K.O. POWER

WORKOUT BLUEPRINT AND TRAINING LOG

BY MARK GINTHER

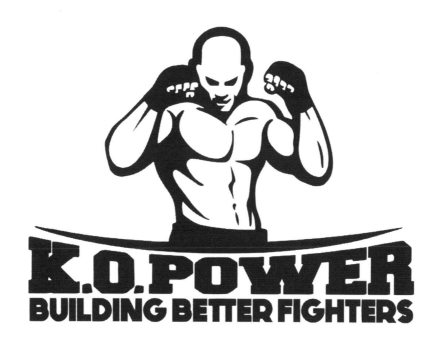

K.O. POWER
WORKOUT BLUEPRINT AND TRAINING LOG

BY MARK GINTHER

Copyright © 2018

ISBN 978-1-942790-12-9

Cover by M.R. Paxson

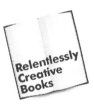

Published by Relentlessly Creative Books
Publisher's Website: http://relentlesslycreativebooks.com/
USA 303-317-2200

TABLE OF CONTENTS

INTRODUCTION

In 2014 I published the book *K.O. Power: Complete Strength Training for Devastating Punches, Kicks, and Throws,* which was the culmination of my (at that time) 15 years professional experience as trainer and coach. Since that time *K.O. Power* has spent over a year on Amazon's best-seller list for Boxing, climbing as high as #2 on the rankings. It has also reached the top ten in Mixed Martial Arts. However, despite its sales record, and favorable reviews, there are those that have difficulty putting the information to practical use.

With those people in mind I have put together the *K.O. Power Workout Blueprint and Training Log,* which has grown out of supplemental materials I have put together for workshops I teach on the subject, to help bridge the gap between theory and application.

This workbook, like most manuals of this kind, is designed to be used with a primary text, in this case, *K.O. Power.* But unlike, for instance, the typical math workbook, which are primarily composed of sample problems corresponding to the materials covered in the various chapters, this workbook is a practical, step-by-step guide that takes you, the reader/user, through what is needed to put together your own training program. It helps you design and customize a program for your specific needs.

In part, the Blueprint is a digest of the material presented *K.O. Power.* But you'll also find a checklist, template and worksheet and training log, which you fill out using the principles introduced in

K.O. Power. It is designed as a tool to augment *K.O. Power,* and is most effective when used with *K.O. Power* as a reference. But the blueprint can work on its own, particularly if you have some previous experience with training concepts such as: maximal strength, explosive power, periodization, macrocycle, etc.

In addition, there is some supplemental material, not covered in *K.O. Power,* and published here for the first time.

WORKOUT BLUEPRINT CHECKLIST

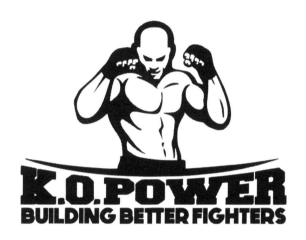

STEP 1: BEGIN WITH THE END IN MIND

First decide on your primary training goal. The primary goal means: Which motor ability is to be the priority in your development? For those whose goal is developing knockout punches and kicks, or lightening takedowns and devastating throws, the goal will be developing explosive power as well as great speed. (For greater detail into the specifics of the relevant motor abilities refer to *K.O. Power,* Chapter II.)

Also, consider your individual strengths and weaknesses. Number them, including both strengths and weaknesses, from 1 to 10, from the most important to the least. It may be necessary to revise this list after completing the testing in Step #2.

Below is a list of motor abilities. Following the description of the motor ability you'll see information about the type of athlete or techniques that ability is an important prerequisite for.

That's not to say that the motor abilities are important for only those attributes listed. It's just that those attributes are prime examples of the applications of such motor abilities. Also included are the primary training protocols to develop each of those motor abilities.

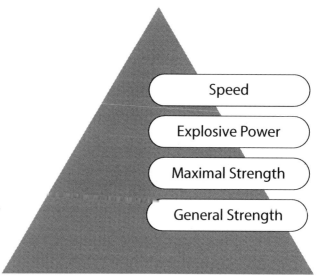

A single training program cannot cover all training goals. But start by choosing a single motor ability as your primary training goal and then add 2 or 3 complimentary and/or prerequisite motor abilities. (See *K.O. Power*, Chapter II for more specifics.}

LIST OF MOTOR ABILITIES:

☑ **Maximal strength:** the amount of musculoskeletal force that can be generated in a single, all-out effort. This is an important prerequisite to all of the other motor abilities listed. (See *K.O. Power*, page 63.)

> **All:** Maximal strength is a prerequisite for all other motor abilities.

> Best developed using loads of 85% 1RM or greater for sets of 5 repetitions for fewer. Greatest results using 90% 1RM or greater for sets of 3 or fewer.

☐ **Strength endurance:** the ability to exert maximal force repeatedly.

> **Grappling:** Moderate loads, 65-85% 1RM for 15-30 repetitions

☐ **Static strength:** the ability to resist force to maintain position.

> **Grappling:** Isometric holds for 15-60 seconds; slow eccentric movements (negatives).

☑ **Relative strength:** one's strength in relation to bodyweight.

> **All:** Especially those competing in a specific weight division. Maximal strength protocols.

☐ **Explosive Power:** A combination of maximal strength and speed. (See *K.O. Power*, page 65.)

> **Grappling:** Movements like suplexes and other similar full-body throws.)

> Best developed using moderate loads of 65-85% moved as quickly as possible for repetitions of 5 or fewer. Modified Olympic lifts are ideally suited for this goal.

☐ **Starting power:** requires the ability to generate maximum force at the onset of a muscular contraction and to achieve a high initial speed.

> **All:** Explosive power protocols.

☐ **Reactive power:** related to reactive strength, the ability to generate force immediately following a landing or after receiving/absorbing force.

> **All:** Stretch-shortening cycle (plyometric drills).

☐ **Power-endurance:** the ability to generate a high degree of power repeatedly.

> **All:** Moderate loads, 50-70% 1RM for 15-30 repetitions

☐ **Strength-speed:** A combination of strength and speed exemplified by movements with rough physical contact.

> **Grappling:** Combination Maximal strength, Explosive power, Reactive power protocols.

☐ **Speed-strength:** A combination of speed and strength exemplified by movements where the body is propelled forward.

> **Grappling:** Shooting; takedowns.

> **Striking:** Heavy kicks and punches, such as shovel hooks. Combination Maximal strength, Explosive power, Reactive power protocols.

☐ **Speed:** The ability to achieve high velocity movement.

> **Striking:** Fast punches and kicks like jabs or snapping kicks. Combination Maximal strength, Explosive power protocols, combined with high-speed ballistic drills.

(Sample routines focusing on the above motor abilities can be found in *K.O. Power,* Chapter X.)

STEP 2: SELF-ASSESSMENT/IDENTIFYING DEFICIENCIES

Consider your 'training age.' How many years have you been engaged in focused strength training? Choose appropriate methods for achieving maximum muscle tension in the targeted muscle groups:

A) The **maximal-effort method** in which one lifts a maximal load.

B) The **repeated-effort method** in which one lifts a sub-maximal load to failure (the final repetitions developing the maximum force possible in a fatigued state).

C) The **dynamic-effort method**, in which one lifts a non-maximal load with the highest speed possible.

These methods will all be used to varying degrees depending on training goals, training age and individual strengths and weaknesses. In a typical, linear training progression, the early phases of training will rely primarily on the repeated-effort method, shifting as the program continues through the progressive phases to maximal-effort and dynamic effort.

For those with less than 3 years of solid, focused training, the repeated-effort method will be primarily used. (See *K.O. Power,* Chapter II for more detail.)

Using test results of 1RM (**1-rep maximum**) in squat, deadlift, and bench press, vertical jump, vertical jump with counter-swing, bench press-throw, etc., determine the weaknesses that must be addressed to meet the final training objective. (See Chapter VI, *K.O. Power* for testing protocols and insert results into table below.)

Exercise			
1RM Tests	1 RM Tested	1RM Estimated	No. Reps Performed at 85% of 1RM
Squat			
Deadlift			
Bench Press			
Power Tests	Static	w/Counter-movement	% Difference
Vertical Jump			
Loaded Jumps/Throws	Weight	Height/Distance	% Difference
Squat Jump (w/vest or barbell)			
Bench-Press Throw			
Seated Shotput-Throw			

PERIODIZATION MODELS

Classical (Linear) Periodization Model

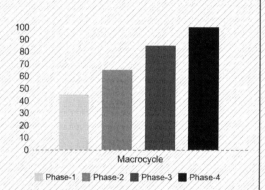

Macrocycle

Phase-1　Phase-2　Phase-3　Phase-4

In a Classical model, loads are increased in a linear, progressive manner from phase (mesocyle) to phase.

Undulating (Alternating) Periodization Model

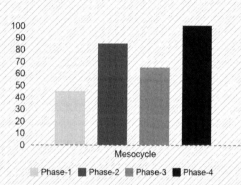

Mesocycle

Phase-1　Phase-2　Phase-3　Phase-4

In a Undulating model, loads are wave loaded in an undulating manner from phase (mesocycle) to phase.

Concurrent (Congugate) Periodization Model

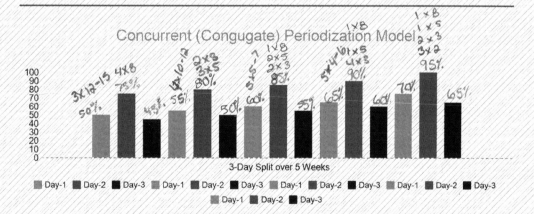

3-Day Split over 5 Weeks

Day-1　Day-2　Day-3　Day-1　Day-2　Day-3　Day-1　Day-2　Day-3　Day-1　Day-2　Day-3

Day-1　Day-2　Day-3

In a Concurrent model, loads will vary in intensity within a given phase (mesocycle), however is still progressive and can be framed within a Classical or Undulating framework.

The Y axis on the charts represents % of 1RM (1 rep maximum).

STEP 3: CHOOSE YOUR TIME FRAME

Choose whether to use a 16-week, 12-week or 8-week plan. Longer cycles are better suited to the novice or those who require remedial training (injury prevention, etc.). An 8-week 'training camp' can also be incorporated into longer 12-16 week plans.

☐ **8 Weeks:** Short, peaking phase. Duration of a typical training camp. Best used to bring together and fine-tune all previous training to peak for competition.

☑ **12 Weeks:** Duration typically required for going from a detrained state to competition ready. Allows enough time to bring up weak areas identified in previous macrocycles.

☐ **16 Weeks:** Longer duration for both 'in-season' (accumulation) and 'pre-season' accentuation training. Good for novices, or for those coming off injuries or other setbacks.

STEP 4: FORMULATE YOUR PLAN

Once you've decided on the number of weeks, divide the weeks into phases of between 2 to 4 weeks. The length of each phase will depend on length of overall program (shorter programs require shorter phases), training age (more advanced lifters adapt faster and therefore do better with shorter phases), and physio-type (stamina types do better on with longer phases, etc.)

Go back to Step- 1, where you numbered the various motor abilities in order of priority. Work backwards from the competition date, starting with the end goal, and progressing to the starting point, considering which motor abilities must be developed to reach the training target. (e.g. maximal strength is a prerequisite for explosive power; general strength a prerequisite for maximal strength, etc.)

STEP 5: FRAME YOUR PLAN

Decide on a periodization model: linear (classical), alternating or concurrent (AKA conjugate).

The classical model is best suited to those who haven't used a periodized plan before. Typically, in a standard, Classical periodized plan, one uses clearly delineated phases, progressing from Anatomical Adaptation (training to train) through Maximal Strength (neuromuscular efficiency) to Explosive Power (increased rate of force development) in a linear (steps 1, 2, 3, 4) progression, relying largely on the Repeated Effort method, transitioning to the Maximal Effort method and on to the Dynamic Effort method.

In an Alternating plan, the progression would be more of an undulating wave than a straightforward, linear progression (steps 1, **3**, 2, **4**).

In a Concurrent plan the Repeated Effort, Maximal Effort and Dynamic Effort methods are all used within the same phase, however it is still progressive, and can be framed within a Classical or Alternating framework. (See Chapter 4, *K.O. Power.*)

STEP 6: ORGANIZE YOUR PLAN

Decide on the duration of each mesocycle. : 2-, 3-, or 4-week cycles. This may be subject to change throughout the program as some motor abilities will require more time/work than others. As mentioned above, 2-week cycles are best for those that are highly trained, as they will adapt more quickly to a given routine, as well as for those that are of the Variable physio type. 4-week cycles are best suited to relative novices, as well as those of the Stamina physio type. 3-week cycles will be appropriate for most, however an 8-week plan demands shorter cycles. A program should have at least 4 phases, but could have as many as 6. Longer programs with shorter cycles would require more total phases.

After considering the criteria in Steps 4-6, choose 1 primary and up to 2 auxiliary motor abilities, as well as the number of weeks per training phase (mesocycle), and write them in the forms as in the example below. Phases do not have to necessarily all be equal in length, particularly in the longer macrocycles.

Example:

12 WEEKS – 2-4 WEEK PHASES (TYPICAL LENGTH 3 WEEKS) 4-6 TOTAL PHASES

Phase-1 *(3 weeks) Primary – Work Capacity· Aux – Joint Stability, Hypertrophy*

Phase-2 *(3 weeks) Primary – Maximal Strength· Aux – Hypertrophy, Joint Stability*

Phase-3 *(2 weeks) Primary – Explosive Power· Aux – Maximal Strength*

Phase-4 *(2 weeks) Primary – Explosive Power· Aux – Strength-Speed*

Phase-5 *(2 weeks) Primary – Speed, Aux – Speed-Strength*

Phase-6 *(1 week) Technical/Tactical Training Only*

8 WEEKS – 2-WEEK PHASES 4 TOTAL PHASES

Phase-1 _____

Phase-2 _____

Phase-3 _____

Phase-4 _____

12 WEEKS – 2-4 WEEK PHASES (TYPICAL LENGTH 3 WEEKS) 4-6 TOTAL PHASES

Phase-1 _____

Phase-2 _____

Phase-3 _____

Phase-4 _____

Phase-5 _____

Phase-6 _____

16 WEEKS – 2-4 WEEKS PHASES (TYPICAL LENGTH 4 WEEKS) 4-6 TOTAL PHASES

Phase-1 _____

Phase-2 _____

Phase-3 _____

Phase-4 _____

Phase-5 _____

Phase-6 _____

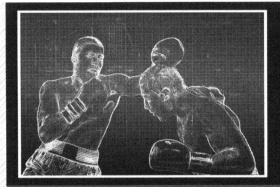

TRAINING THE ENERGY PATHWAYS:

The Three Primary Modes of Endurance Training

A proper framework is needed to manage the various training adaptations in a way that facilitates the effective development of each characteristic

Long, Slow Distance Training (LSD)	Lower-Intensity Interval Training (LIIT)	High-Intensity Interval Training (HIIT)
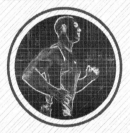	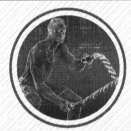	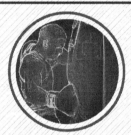

PRIORITIZATION AND INTEGRATION

The various endurance training modalities should not be used haphazardly or indiscriminately, but must be balanced with technical, tactical and strength training.

LSD (Slow-Twitch Aerobic Fibers) Characterized by slow, long duration, steady-state exercises like distance running, rowing, cycling, etc.

Non-specific to the intermittent nature of most fight sports. Can be used (if at all) during 'active rest' periods, or for untrained individuals to build an 'aerobic base'.

LIIT (Intermediary & Fast-Twitch Fibers) Characterized by lower-impact movements (rope skipping, rhythmic battle-rope drills, shadow boxing, etc.) performed for up to 60 seconds.

Suggested 1:1 work-to-rest ratio, applied during early phases of training; paired with higher-volume resistance training (e.g. Anatomical Adaptation; Hypertrophy training).

HIIT (Fast-Twitch Fibers) Characterized by high-speed, high-intensity movements (bag work, sprints, burpees, etc.) performed all-out for 10-15 seconds.

Suggested 1:2 work-to-rest ratio, applied following earlier phases of training; paired with strength and strength-power training for the remainder of the cycle.

STEP 7: CHART YOUR COURSE

Plot the program onto the timeline in the worksheets at the bottom as in the examples below. The first example depicts a linear model using 3-week mesocycles. The second example is of an alternating model using 2-week mesocycles. The alternating structure and shorter cycles are well suited to more finely tuned adaptations.

Week 1	Week 2	Week 3	Week 4	Week 5	Week 6	Week 7	Week 8	Week 9	Week 10	Week 11	Week 12
Anatomical Adaption Reps, 8-12RM			General Strength Reps, 6-8RM			Maximal Strength Reps, 1-RM			Conversion to Power Reps, 4-8 @ 65-8% 1RM		

Week 1	Week 2	Week 3	Week 4	Week 5	Week 6	Week 7	Week 8	Week 9	Week 10	Week 11	Week 12
General Strength Reps, 5-7		Strength- Speed Reps, 2-4		Maximal Strengths Reps, 1-4		Speed Strength Reps, 5-7		Explosive Power Reps, 4-6		Speed/Taper Reps, 6-8	

A concurrent program, where *Maximal Effort, Dynamic Effort* and *Repetitive Effort* are all trained within a week could be fit into either a linear or alternating framework; the volume and intensity of each training day being dictated by the phase. (Note: Unlike the examples, phases do not necessarily need to be of the same duration; more or less time may be allocated to a phase depending on needs.)

STEP 8: PRIORITIZE, DIVIDE AND ASSIGN

Next you'll have to decide how many days to split training into, 2, 3 or 4 (4 days best when strength training is the priority, 3 for most other cases, and 2 days when tapering for competition or for maintenance), which days to perform strength training, how to schedule it (avoid the same movement patterns and/or loads in consecutive workouts) with other training, technical and tactical.

Ideally strength training should be performed 4 to 6 hours apart from technical training, but this often is not realistic with work schedules and such. If they must be performed in the same session, strength training should follow skill training. Also, technical, strength and endurance training need not be entirely separate spheres, but can and do overlap (the degree will vary according to the training phase). For example: Anaerobic punching intervals on a heavybag could be considered strength training (dynamic strength), endurance (anaerobic-phosphate) and technical (punching technique).

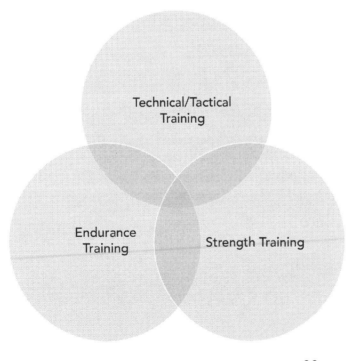

Following is an example using a 3-day split, using full-body workouts in a concurrent periodization scheme. Also in the example below are suggestions for scheduling other training demands.

Week-1						
M	T	W	T	F	S	S
12pm Skill Training 6pm Strength Training—Dynamic Effort	12pm Skill Training followed by conditioning drills on heavy bag or pads	12pm Skill Training 6pm Strength Training—Maximal Effort	12pm Skill Training followed by conditioning drills on heavy bag or pads	12pm Sparring 6pm Strength/Conditioning combined training—Repetitive Effort	Off	Off

STEP 9: ORGANIZE AND DIVIDE

Decide how to split the movements. For athletic training, unlike bodybuilding, semi full-body training (or upper-body, lower-body splits) is recommended.   Balance pushing and pulling movements, both within each workout and within each phase. Avoid training the same movement patterns and/or loads in consecutive training sessions.

STEP 10: PRESCRIBE

Once the starting phase is determined, choose appropriate exercises (e.g. unilateral movements are best suited to Anatomical Adaptation; compound, multi-joint movements like deadlift best suited to Maximal Strength), and set and rep schemes.

Following are some examples of exercises organized by suited training objective. Note: These exercises need not need to be used exclusively for the listed training objective. These examples represent their typical use. (See *K.O. Power*, Chapter 9 for a more complete list (and detailed explanations).)

Anatomical Adaptation (prehabilitation): These exercises are typically characterized as being unilateral (single-limbed), often single-jointed, using a relatively small load (40-60% 1RM), as well as often requiring greater balance and joint stability. Many of these exercises, when using greater loads can be well suited to developing general strength as well.

> lunges
> step-ups
> side-press
> external rotations
> Cuban presses
> calf raises
> windmills
> wrist curls
> sit-throughs

Maximal Strength (neuromuscular efficiency): These exercises are characterized as being multi-jointed (or even full-body), bilateral (using both limbs), and using great loads (heavy resistance 85-100% 1RM). Many of these exercises can be used effectively with more moderate loads for developing general strength.

squat
deadlift
bench press
dips
overhead press

Explosive Power (increased rate of force production): These exercises are characterized by rapid execution, close to or reaching sport-speed, and include modified Olympic lifts, plyometrics, and ballistic movements. Some, like power cleans, are best used for developing power on the force end of the force-speed spectrum (65-85% 1RM), while others, like medicine-ball passes, are better for developing the speed end of the spectrum (see *K.O. Power*, Chapter 2).

That said, many of the movements can be adjusted toward either end of the spectrum simply by adjusting the loading parameters: Lighter weight, higher speed of execution. Heavier weight, greater development of force.

power clean
power snatch
kettlebell swing
medicine ball passes
box jumps

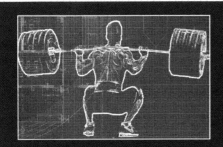

PRIMARY STRENGTH TRAINING METHODS:

REPEATED EFFORT
MAXIMAL EFFORT
DYNAMIC EFFORT

 THERE ARE THREE PRIMARY TRAINING METHODS FOR CREATING MAXIMAL TENSION IN THE WORKING MUSCLES.

1. REPEATED EFFORT	2. MAXIMAL EFFORT	3. DYNAMIC EFFORT
A sub-maximal load is lifted till near muscular failure, developing maximal force in a fatigued state.	 A maximal or near-maximal load is lifted.	 A non-maximal load is lifted with the highest speeds possible.
Appropriate for Anatomical Adaptation and General Strength phases.	Appropriate for Maximal Strength and Explosive Power phases.	Appropriate for Explosive Power and Speed phases.

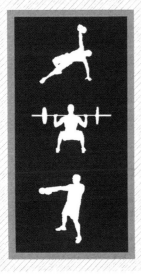

1. Best achieved with unilateral movements and those focusing on range of motion and mobility, such as lunges, step-ups full squats, side-presses, sit-thrus, gymnastics inspired movements, and such.

2. Best achieved with bilateral, multi-joint movements, such as squat, deadlift, bench press, bar dips, pull-ups, and such.

3. Best achieved with explosive, high-speed movements such as plyometrics, modified Olympic lifts, kettlebell swings, medicine ball passes, and such.

A typical Anatomical Adaptation workout to correct muscular imbalances and strengthen weak links might look like the following.

Anatomical Adaptation (full body): Day-1				
Exercise	Weight	Sets	Repetitions	Rest Interval
Reverse Lunge w/dumbbells	30lbs each hand	2	24 (alternating, 12per leg)	1 min
Single-leg Semi-Stiff Legged Deadlift w/dumbbells	30lbs each hand	2, 1 set per leg	10	1 min
Mixed Grip Chins	Bodyweight	2, 1 set per hand position	12	2 min
Incline Dumbbell Press	45lbs	2	10, alternating, 5 per arm	90 seconds
Cuban Press w/dumbbells	25lbs	2	8	90 seconds
Russian Twists w/dumbbell	15lbs	2	16	1 min
Single-Leg Lying Hip/ Thigh Extension	Bodyweight	2	20, alternating, 10 per leg	1 min
Single-leg Calf Raise w/dumbbell	60lbs	4, 2 per leg	8	30 seconds

A typical Maximal Strength workout might look like the following chart. As you can see, the greater the intensity (based on percentage of 1RM), the lower the volume of training). (See *K.O. Power*, Chapter III for more information.)

Maximal Strength (full body): Day-1

Exercise	Weight	Sets	Repetitions	Rest Interval
Deadlift	360lbs	3	3	5 min
Barbell Floor Press	245lbs	3	3	5 min
Saxon Side Bend w/dumbbells	10lbs each dumbbell	3	8	2 min

A typical program power for Explosive Power might look like this:

Explosive Power (full body): Day-1

Exercise	Weight	Sets	Repetitions	Rest Interval
Power Cleans	135lbs	3-4	4-6	3 min
Push-Jerk	135lbs	2-3	2-4	1 min
Explosive Chins	Bodyweight	2	4-6	2 min
Medicine-Ball Pass	20bs	2	6-8	90 seconds
Russian Twists w/medicine ball	20lbs	2	16-20	1 min

STEP 11: MAP IT OUT

Considering the criteria above and following the examples, fill out the following forms either using the 8, 12 or 16-week box. Draw your own vertical lines (as in the example in step 7). Once the overall plan is mapped out, and the protocols for the starting phase determined, you are ready to begin.

LONG-TERM PLANNING: MACROCYCLE AND MESOCYCLES

Week 1	Week 2	Week 3	Week 4	Week 5	Week 6	Week 7	Week 8

Week 1	Week 2	Week 3	Week 4	Week 5	Week 6	Week 7	Week 8	Week 9	Week 10	Week 11	Week 12

Wk 1	Wk 2	Wk 3	Wk 4	Wk 5	Wk 6	Wk 7	Wk 8	Wk 9	Wk 10	Wk 11	Wk 12	Wk 13	Wk 14	Wk 15	Wk 16

STEP 12: REVISE AND AMEND

The plan is not meant to be iron-clad, but flexible, and revised as necessary. A workout log will need to be kept, and progress charted. The phases may be lengthened or shortened depending on progress. Recovery periods may need to be worked in between phases. This can be done by either reducing the volume (number of sets and exercises per workout), or by taking extra recovery days. The flow chart below shows how you may review and rework your plan following each phase of the program.

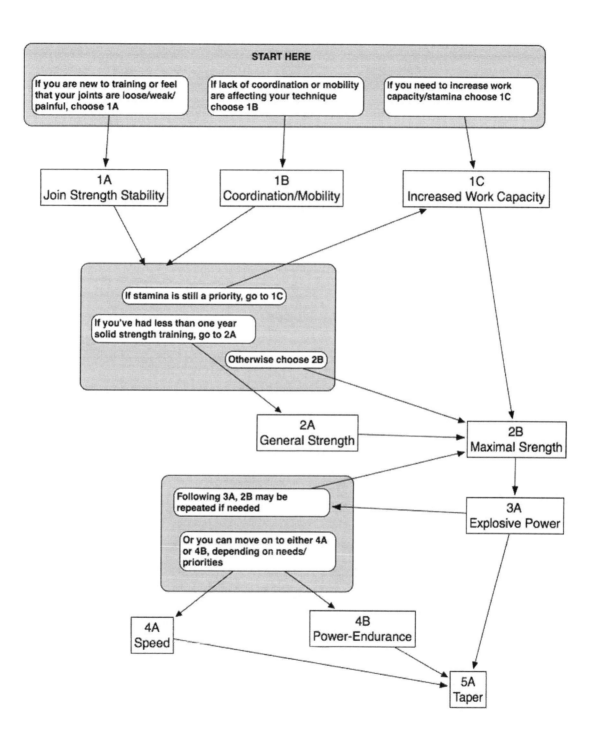

MICROCYCLES: WEEKLY AND DAILY PLANNING

Progression: Training needs to be progressive from week to week. This can be done by either increasing weight, increasing number of repetitions, decreasing the rest intervals, or some combination of these.

Endurance: When endurance is the goal, work to decrease rest intervals and increase reps and sets. But don't try to do all at once. Decreasing rest intervals is best when trying to improve recovery ability. Increasing sets when the goal maintain performance level for greater duration. Increase sets when the goal is to increase the number of exertions you can perform in a single effort (as in a barrage of punches or kicks).

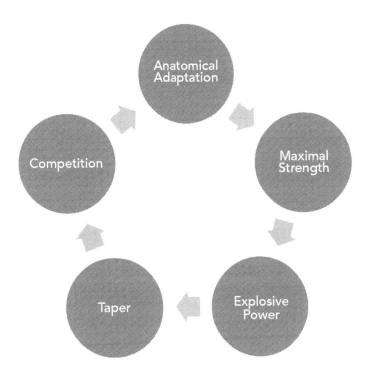

Maximal Strength: When increasing absolute or relative strength, increase load each week rather than number of sets.

Explosive Power: When increasing explosive power is the goal, increase load each subsequent week of a given workout. For power-endurance, increase the number of reps or sets, or decrease length of rest intervals following the protocols above.

Taper: When tapering for competition reduce training volume (number of days trained per week, number of total sets performed per workout), not intensity (as measured by % of 1RM).

Below are forms to plan your weekly training as in the examples above. There are forms enough for up to a 16-week program. I don't recommend filling out the entire program by week (you have your long-term planning mapped out above), but rather do it week by week, keeping it flexible and subject to change.

Following the weekly forms are forms for daily training. Sufficient forms for 16 weeks of 3xWeek training is provided. Again, don't fill out more than 1 week at a time—3 sheet per week for most people in most phases. Use the space provided for notes keeping track of things like whether the resistance and volume felt right, levels of energy or fatigue and such.

Following each week assess progress, troubleshoot any problems or difficulties, referring to the steps above and *K.O. Power: Complete Strength Training for Devastating Punches, Kicks, and Throws.* Make adjustments as needed and continue. Following each phase, do the same before deciding on the exact weekly and daily plans.

K.O. POWER TRAINING LOG

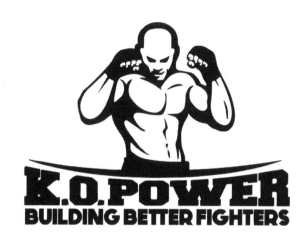

TRAINING LOG

The following training log can accommodate up to a 16 week program, set up for a 5-day split strength training regimen. Below are examples of how to fill out both the weekly and daily planning forms.

WEEKLY PLANNING

The weekly planning forms are comprised of both a weekly calendar designed for scheduling training days, times and methods, and a form for individually listing and detailing the specific training modalities, such as, aerobic, anaerobic, resistance and technical/tactical training.

The example below shows hypothetical scheduling of a training regimen for a MMA fighter that may also works a full-time job, requiring training be in a single block. This is not optimal, but often a reality. A professional fighter, with no additional commitments could (and should) divide his/her training into separate AM/PM blocks, optimally 4 to 6 hours apart.

Week						
M	**T**	**W**	**T**	**F**	**S**	**S**
6pm: Striking	6pm: Grappling	6pm: Striking	6pm: Grappling	6pm: MMA	Off	Off
8pm: Strength Training	8pm Heavybag Intervals	8pm: Strength Training	8pm: Dummy Throws, rounds	8pm: Strength Training		

Note that in the example, an attempt is made to balance the various training modalities, striking/grappling, strength/endurance, technical/tactical, etc. The plan need not be set in stone, but should be flexible, and open to change.

In the form below is an example of how to record the individual training modalities according to their function, and primary energy pathway.

Note that there is no specifically aerobic drills (though many of the other drills will contain an aerobic component. See *K.O. Power*, Chapter V.) As the focus of this training phase is Conversion to Power, a phase fairly late in the program, endurance training will be primarily anaerobic in nature.

Training Modality	Method, Duration, Focus, Day(s)
Technical/Tactical	*MON: Counter-Punching Drills. Sparring.* *TUE: Submissions. Rolling.* *WED: Punch/Kick Combos. Sparring.* *FRI: Sparring*
Anaerobic	*TUE: Heavybag Intervals – 3, 5 min rounds* *THU: Dummy Throws – 3, 5 min rounds*
Aerobic	
Resistance	*MON: Plyometric & Ballistic Drills. 45 min.* *WED: Power Clean and Push-Press. 60 min.* *FRI: Dynamic Circuit. 30 min.*

To avoid undue redundancy in training (which can result in over-training), keep in mind that in many cases there will be overlap in the training adaptations of the various drills. For example: The counter-punching drills that are listed as Technical/Tactical, will also (depending on intensity of practice) will also require Endurance capabilities. And, rolling (grappling sparring) will require combine elements of Strength and Endurance with Technical and Tactical work.

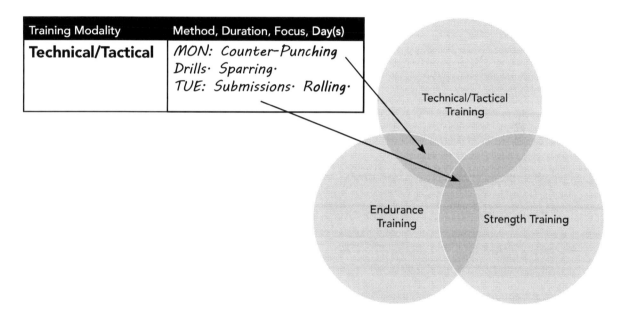

Training Modality	Method, Duration, Focus, Day(s)
Technical/Tactical	*MON: Counter-Punching Drills. Sparring. TUE: Submissions. Rolling.*

Both the weekly and daily planning sections have space for personal notes. These can be used for record anything that stands out: Deviations from planning, thoughts/plans for upcoming sessions and the like.

"I was able to convince my body that I could take it and nobody could hurt me. I might've gotten cut, stitches over my eyes. Broken nose. Broken hands. But I never really got hurt."
—Jake LaMotta

DAILY PLANNING: INDIVIDUAL WORKOUTS

Training Adaptation ___Max Strength___   Training Day ___Day-2, Max-Effort___

Exercise	Weight	Sets	Repetitions	Rest Interval
Back Squat, medium stance, below parallel	315lbs	3	3 (2 on last set)	4 min
Back (1/4) Squats, medium stance, above parallel·	385lbs	1	3	4 min
Overhead Barbell Press from chest	165lbs	3	3	2 min
Superset w/Underhand Weighted Chins medium grip	Body-weight+ 55lbs	3	3	2 min
Overhead Barbell Press from pins (1/4 range)	185lbs	1	3	2 min
Superset w/Underhand Weighted Chins medium grip, negative reps	Body-weight+ 75lbs	1	1 w/15 sec hold, and 15 sec descent	4 min
Saxon Side-Bend w/dumbbells	15lbs each hand	2	8	2 min

Notes   Was unable to get final rep on last set of squats· Probably residu-al fatigue from previous cardio session· Will back off on next cardio session and keep weights same in squats next week· Will try to add 5% on other lifts· Don't forget chalk next time·

LONG-TERM PLANNING: MACROCYCLE AND MESOCYCLES

Week 1	Week 2	Week 3	Week 4	Week 5	Week 6	Week 7	Week 8

Week 1	Week 2	Week 3	Week 4	Week 5	Week 6	Week 7	Week 8	Week 9	Week 10	Week 11	Week 12

Wk 1	Wk 2	Wk 3	Wk 4	Wk 5	Wk 6	Wk 7	Wk 8	Wk 9	Wk 10	Wk 11	Wk 12	Wk 13	Wk 14	Wk 15	Wk 16

LONG-TERM PLANNING: MACROCYCLE AND MESOCYCLES

Week 1	Week 2	Week 3	Week 4	Week 5	Week 6	Week 7	Week 8

Week 1	Week 2	Week 3	Week 4	Week 5	Week 6	Week 7	Week 8	Week 9	Week 10	Week 11	Week 12

Wk 1	Wk 2	Wk 3	Wk 4	Wk 5	Wk 6	Wk 7	Wk 8	Wk 9	Wk 10	Wk 11	Wk 12	Wk 13	Wk 14	Wk 15	Wk 16

Weekly Training

Training Phase _____

Mon	Tue	Wed	Thur	Fri	Sat	Sun

Training Modality	Method, Duration, Focus, Day(s)
Technical/Tactical	
Anaerobic	
Aerobic	
Resistance	

Notes

_____

_____

_____

_____

"Today is victory over yourself of yesterday;
tomorrow is victory over lesser men."
—*Miyamoto Musashi*

DAILY PLANNING: INDIVIDUAL WORKOUTS

Training Adaptation _____   Training Day_____

Exercise	Weight	Sets	Repetitions	Rest Interval

Notes _____

_____

_____

"Accept the challenges so that you may feel
the exhilaration of victory."
—George Patton

DAILY PLANNING: INDIVIDUAL WORKOUTS

Training Adaptation _____ Training Day_____

Exercise	Weight	Sets	Repetitions	Rest Interval

Notes
_____
_____
_____
_____

*"By forgetting the past and by throwing myself into
other interests, I forget to worry."*
—Jack Dempsey

DAILY PLANNING: INDIVIDUAL WORKOUTS

Training Adaptation _____   Training Day_____

Exercise	Weight	Sets	Repetitions	Rest Interval

Notes _____

_____

_____

"Discipline in war counts more than fury."

—*Niccolo Machiavelli*

DAILY PLANNING: INDIVIDUAL WORKOUTS

Training Adaptation _____   Training Day_____

Exercise	Weight	Sets	Repetitions	Rest Interval

Notes _____

_____

_____

_____

"In every battle there is a time when both sides consider themselves beaten, then he who continues the attack wins."
—Ulysses S. Grant

DAILY PLANNING: INDIVIDUAL WORKOUTS

Training Adaptation _____ Training Day_____

Exercise	Weight	Sets	Repetitions	Rest Interval

Notes
_____
_____
_____

Weekly Training

Training Phase _____

Mon	Tue	Wed	Thur	Fri	Sat	Sun

Training Modality	Method, Duration, Focus, Day(s)
Technical/Tactical	
Anaerobic	
Aerobic	
Resistance	

Notes

_____

_____

_____

_____

"There are no limits. There are plateaus, but you must not stay there, you must go beyond them."
—Bruce Lee

DAILY PLANNING: INDIVIDUAL WORKOUTS

Training Adaptation _____   Training Day_____

Exercise	Weight	Sets	Repetitions	Rest Interval

Notes _____

_____

_____

_____

"You can map out a fight plan or a life plan, but when the action starts, it may not go the way you planned, and you're down to your reflexes—that means your [preparation]."
—Joe Frazier

DAILY PLANNING: INDIVIDUAL WORKOUTS

Training Adaptation _____ Training Day_____

Exercise	Weight	Sets	Repetitions	Rest Interval

Notes
_____
_____
_____
_____

"In preparing for battle I have always found that plans
are useless, but planning essential."
—Dwight D. Eisenhower

DAILY PLANNING: INDIVIDUAL WORKOUTS

Training Adaptation _____   Training Day _____

Exercise	Weight	Sets	Repetitions	Rest Interval

Notes _____

_____

_____

_____

"Through every generation there has been a constant war, a war with fear. Those who have the courage to conquer fear are made free; those that are conquered by it are made to suffer until they have the courage to defeat it, or death takes them."
—Alexander the Great

DAILY PLANNING: INDIVIDUAL WORKOUTS

Training Adaptation _____   Training Day_____

Exercise	Weight	Sets	Repetitions	Rest Interval

Notes
_____
_____
_____
_____

"Courage—a perfect sensibility of the measure of danger and the mental willingness to endure it."
—William Tecumseh Sherman

DAILY PLANNING: INDIVIDUAL WORKOUTS

Training Adaptation _____   Training Day_____

Exercise	Weight	Sets	Repetitions	Rest Interval

Notes

_____

_____

_____

Weekly Training

Training Phase _____

Mon	Tue	Wed	Thur	Fri	Sat	Sun

Training Modality	Method, Duration, Focus, Day(s)
Technical/Tactical	
Anaerobic	
Aerobic	
Resistance	

Notes

_____

_____

_____

_____

"I will either find a way, or I will make one."

—Hannibal

DAILY PLANNING: INDIVIDUAL WORKOUTS

Training Adaptation _____   Training Day_____

Exercise	Weight	Sets	Repetitions	Rest Interval

Notes _____

_____

_____

_____

"It is easier to find men willing to volunteer to die, than to find those that are willing to endure pain with patience."
—Julius Caesar

DAILY PLANNING: INDIVIDUAL WORKOUTS

Training Adaptation _____ Training Day _____

Exercise	Weight	Sets	Repetitions	Rest Interval

Notes _____

_____

_____

_____

"Sure the fight was fixed. I fixed it with a right hand."

—George Foreman

DAILY PLANNING: INDIVIDUAL WORKOUTS

Training Adaptation _____ Training Day_____

Exercise	Weight	Sets	Repetitions	Rest Interval

Notes
_____
_____
_____

"Fast is fine, but accuracy is everything."

—Xenophon

DAILY PLANNING: INDIVIDUAL WORKOUTS

Training Adaptation _____ Training Day_____

Exercise	Weight	Sets	Repetitions	Rest Interval

Notes _____

_____

_____

"In battle, if you make your opponent flinch, you have already won."

—*Miyamoto Musashi*

DAILY PLANNING: INDIVIDUAL WORKOUTS

Training Adaptation _____ Training Day_____

Exercise	Weight	Sets	Repetitions	Rest Interval

Notes

_____

_____

_____

Weekly Training

Training Phase _____

Mon	Tue	Wed	Thur	Fri	Sat	Sun

Training Modality	Method, Duration, Focus, Day(s)
Technical/Tactical	
Anaerobic	
Aerobic	
Resistance	

Notes

_____

_____

_____

_____

"One must therefore be a fox to recognize traps, and a lion to frighten wolves. Those that only wish to be lions do not understand this."
—Niccolo Machiavelli

DAILY PLANNING: INDIVIDUAL WORKOUTS

Training Adaptation _____ Training Day_____

Exercise	Weight	Sets	Repetitions	Rest Interval

Notes _____

_____

_____

_____

"It is fatal to enter into any war without the will to win it."

—*Douglas MacArthur*

DAILY PLANNING: INDIVIDUAL WORKOUTS

Training Adaptation _____ Training Day_____

Exercise	Weight	Sets	Repetitions	Rest Interval

Notes

_____

_____

_____

"It's not the light we need, but the fire; it's not the gentle shower, but thunder. We need the storm, the whirlwind and the earthquake."
—Frederick Douglas

DAILY PLANNING: INDIVIDUAL WORKOUTS

Training Adaptation _____   Training Day_____

Exercise	Weight	Sets	Repetitions	Rest Interval

Notes _____

_____

_____

"Pursue one great decisive aim with force and determination."

—*Carl von Clausewitz*

DAILY PLANNING: INDIVIDUAL WORKOUTS

Training Adaptation _____ Training Day_____

Exercise	Weight	Sets	Repetitions	Rest Interval

Notes _____

_____

_____

_____

"Rules are made to be broken and are too often
for the lazy to hide behind."
—Douglas MacArthur

DAILY PLANNING: INDIVIDUAL WORKOUTS

Training Adaptation _____   Training Day_____

Exercise	Weight	Sets	Repetitions	Rest Interval

Notes _____

_____

_____

Weekly Training

Training Phase _____

Mon	Tue	Wed	Thur	Fri	Sat	Sun

Training Modality	Method, Duration, Focus, Day(s)
Technical/Tactical	
Anaerobic	
Aerobic	
Resistance	

Notes
_____
_____
_____
_____

"If you're going through hell, keep going."

—*Winston Churchill*

DAILY PLANNING: INDIVIDUAL WORKOUTS

Training Adaptation _____ Training Day _____

Exercise	Weight	Sets	Repetitions	Rest Interval

Notes _____

_____

_____

_____

"Do not deny the classical approach, simply as a reaction, or you will have created another pattern and trapped yourself there."
—*Bruce Lee*

DAILY PLANNING: INDIVIDUAL WORKOUTS

Training Adaptation _____   Training Day _____

Exercise	Weight	Sets	Repetitions	Rest Interval

Notes

_____

_____

_____

"Impetuosity and audacity many times can obtain that which, with ordinary means can never be obtained."
—Niccolo Machiavelli

DAILY PLANNING: INDIVIDUAL WORKOUTS

Training Adaptation _____   Training Day_____

Exercise	Weight	Sets	Repetitions	Rest Interval

Notes
_____
_____
_____

"The true science of the martial arts means practicing in such a way
that they will be useful at any time, and to teach them is such
a way that they will be useful in all things."
—*Miyamoto Musashi*

DAILY PLANNING: INDIVIDUAL WORKOUTS

Training Adaptation _____ Training Day_____

Exercise	Weight	Sets	Repetitions	Rest Interval

Notes

_____

_____

_____

_____

"Knowledge and Courage are the elements of Greatness. They give immortality, because they are immortal. Each is as much as he knows, and the wise can do anything. A man without knowledge, a world without light. Wisdom and strength, eyes and hands. Knowledge without courage is sterile." —Baltasar Gracián

DAILY PLANNING: INDIVIDUAL WORKOUTS

Training Adaptation _____   Training Day _____

Exercise	Weight	Sets	Repetitions	Rest Interval

Notes _____

_____

_____

_____

Weekly Training

Training Phase _____

Mon	Tue	Wed	Thur	Fri	Sat	Sun

Training Modality	Method, Duration, Focus, Day(s)
Technical/Tactical	
Anaerobic	
Aerobic	
Resistance	

Notes

_____

_____

_____

_____

"Only sex and sleep make me conscious that I am mortal."

—Alexander the Great

DAILY PLANNING: INDIVIDUAL WORKOUTS

Training Adaptation _____   Training Day_____

Exercise	Weight	Sets	Repetitions	Rest Interval

Notes _____

_____

_____

_____

"The important thing in strategy is to suppress the enemy's useful actions, but to allow his useless actions."
—*Miyamoto Musashi*

DAILY PLANNING: INDIVIDUAL WORKOUTS

Training Adaptation _____   Training Day_____

Exercise	Weight	Sets	Repetitions	Rest Interval

Notes _____
_____
_____
_____

"There is no security on this earth; there is only opportunity."

—*Douglas MacArthur*

DAILY PLANNING: INDIVIDUAL WORKOUTS

Training Adaptation _____   Training Day_____

Exercise	Weight	Sets	Repetitions	Rest Interval

Notes _____

_____

_____

_____

"There are roads which must not be followed, armies which must not be attacked, towns which must not be besieged, positions which must not be contested, commands of the sovereign which must not be obeyed."
—Sun Tzu

DAILY PLANNING: INDIVIDUAL WORKOUTS

Training Adaptation _____   Training Day_____

Exercise	Weight	Sets	Repetitions	Rest Interval

Notes _____

_____

_____

_____

DAILY PLANNING: INDIVIDUAL WORKOUTS

Training Adaptation _____ Training Day _____

Exercise	Weight	Sets	Repetitions	Rest Interval

Notes _____

_____

_____

_____

Weekly Training

Training Phase _____

Mon	Tue	Wed	Thur	Fri	Sat	Sun

Training Modality	Method, Duration, Focus, Day(s)
Technical/Tactical	
Anaerobic	
Aerobic	
Resistance	

Notes

_____

_____

_____

_____

"Our knowledge of circumstances has increased, but our uncertainty, instead of having diminished, has only increased. The reason of this is, that we do not gain all our experience at once, but by degrees; so our determinations continue to be assailed incessantly by fresh experience; and the mind, if we may use the expression, must always be under arms." —Carl von Clausewitz

DAILY PLANNING: INDIVIDUAL WORKOUTS

Training Adaptation _____   Training Day_____

Exercise	Weight	Sets	Repetitions	Rest Interval

Notes
_____
_____
_____

*"Events of future history will be of the same nature—or nearly so—
as the history of the past, so long as men are men."*
—Thucydides

DAILY PLANNING: INDIVIDUAL WORKOUTS

Training Adaptation _____   Training Day_____

Exercise	Weight	Sets	Repetitions	Rest Interval

Notes
_____
_____
_____

"Boxing is like jazz. The better it is, the less people appreciate it."

—*George Foreman*

DAILY PLANNING: INDIVIDUAL WORKOUTS

Training Adaptation _____   Training Day_____

Exercise	Weight	Sets	Repetitions	Rest Interval

Notes
_____
_____
_____

"To know how to recognize an opportunity in war, and to take it,
benefits you more than anything else."
—Niccolo Machiavelli

DAILY PLANNING: INDIVIDUAL WORKOUTS

Training Adaptation _____   Training Day_____

Exercise	Weight	Sets	Repetitions	Rest Interval

Notes
_____
_____
_____

"Do nothing that is of no use."

—*Miyamoto Musashi*

DAILY PLANNING: INDIVIDUAL WORKOUTS

Training Adaptation _____ Training Day_____

Exercise	Weight	Sets	Repetitions	Rest Interval

Notes
_____
_____
_____

Weekly Training

Training Phase _____

Mon	Tue	Wed	Thur	Fri	Sat	Sun

Training Modality	Method, Duration, Focus, Day(s)
Technical/Tactical	
Anaerobic	
Aerobic	
Resistance	

Notes

_____

_____

_____

_____

"We are not retreating, we are advancing in another direction."

—Douglas MacArthur

DAILY PLANNING: INDIVIDUAL WORKOUTS

Training Adaptation _____   Training Day_____

Exercise	Weight	Sets	Repetitions	Rest Interval

Notes
_____
_____
_____

"Glory is fleeting, but obscurity is forever."

—*Napoleon*

DAILY PLANNING: INDIVIDUAL WORKOUTS

Training Adaptation _____   Training Day_____

Exercise	Weight	Sets	Repetitions	Rest Interval

Notes

_____

_____

_____

"[The Spartans] should not make war often, or long, with the same enemy, lest that they should train and instruct them in war, by habituating them to defend themselves."
—Plutarch

DAILY PLANNING: INDIVIDUAL WORKOUTS

Training Adaptation _____   Training Day_____

Exercise	Weight	Sets	Repetitions	Rest Interval

Notes
_____
_____
_____
_____

"Attack is the secret of defense; defense is the planning of an attack."

—*Sun Tzu*

DAILY PLANNING: INDIVIDUAL WORKOUTS

Training Adaptation _____   Training Day_____

Exercise	Weight	Sets	Repetitions	Rest Interval

Notes

_____

_____

_____

"I was able to convince my body that I could take it and nobody could hurt me. I might've gotten cut, stitches over my eyes. Broken nose. Broken hands. But I never really got hurt."
—*Jake LaMotta*

DAILY PLANNING: INDIVIDUAL WORKOUTS

Training Adaptation _____   Training Day_____

Exercise	Weight	Sets	Repetitions	Rest Interval

Notes
_____
_____
_____

Weekly Training

Training Phase _____

Mon	Tue	Wed	Thur	Fri	Sat	Sun

Training Modality	Method, Duration, Focus, Day(s)
Technical/Tactical	
Anaerobic	
Aerobic	
Resistance	

Notes _____

_____

_____

_____

"I prayed for twenty years but received no answer
until I prayed with my legs."
—Frederick Douglas

DAILY PLANNING: INDIVIDUAL WORKOUTS

Training Adaptation _____   Training Day_____

Exercise	Weight	Sets	Repetitions	Rest Interval

Notes

_____

_____

_____

"He who defends everything, defends nothing."

—Frederick the Great

DAILY PLANNING: INDIVIDUAL WORKOUTS

Training Adaptation _____   Training Day_____

Exercise	Weight	Sets	Repetitions	Rest Interval

Notes
_____
_____
_____
_____

"Take time to deliberate, but when the time for action comes,
stop thinking and go in."
—Napoleon

DAILY PLANNING: INDIVIDUAL WORKOUTS

Training Adaptation _____   Training Day_____

Exercise	Weight	Sets	Repetitions	Rest Interval

Notes
_____
_____
_____
_____

"If you're afraid—don't do it; if you're doing it—don't be afraid!"

—Genghis Khan

DAILY PLANNING: INDIVIDUAL WORKOUTS

Training Adaptation _____ Training Day_____

Exercise	Weight	Sets	Repetitions	Rest Interval

Notes _____

_____

_____

_____

"Prepare for the unknown by studying how others in the past have coped for the unforeseeable and the unpredictable."
—George S. Patton

DAILY PLANNING: INDIVIDUAL WORKOUTS

Training Adaptation _____   Training Day _____

Exercise	Weight	Sets	Repetitions	Rest Interval

Notes

_____

_____

_____

Weekly Training

Training Phase _____

Mon	Tue	Wed	Thur	Fri	Sat	Sun

Training Modality	Method, Duration, Focus, Day(s)
Technical/Tactical	
Anaerobic	
Aerobic	
Resistance	

Notes
_____
_____
_____
_____

"The art of war is simple enough. Find out where your enemy is. Get at him as soon as you can. Strike him as hard as you can, and keep moving on."
—Ulysses S. Grant

DAILY PLANNING: INDIVIDUAL WORKOUTS

Training Adaptation _____   Training Day_____

Exercise	Weight	Sets	Repetitions	Rest Interval

Notes
_____
_____
_____

*"The fighter that's gone into the ring and hasn't experienced fear is
either a liar or a psychopath."*
—Cus D'Amato

DAILY PLANNING: INDIVIDUAL WORKOUTS

Training Adaptation _____   Training Day _____

Exercise	Weight	Sets	Repetitions	Rest Interval

Notes _____

_____

_____

_____

"It is not uncommon for fighters' camps to be gloomy. In heavy training, fighters live in dimensions of boredom others do not begin to contemplate. Fighters are supposed to. The boredom creates an impatience with one's life, and a violence to improve it. Boredom creates a detestation for losing." —Norman Mailer

DAILY PLANNING: INDIVIDUAL WORKOUTS

Training Adaptation _____   Training Day_____

Exercise	Weight	Sets	Repetitions	Rest Interval

Notes
_____
_____
_____

"I can entertain the proposition that life is a metaphor for boxing—for one of those bouts that go on and on, round following round, jabs, missed punches, clinches, nothing determined, again the bell and again and you and your opponent so evenly matched it's impossible to see your opponent is you ..." —Joyce Carol Oates

DAILY PLANNING: INDIVIDUAL WORKOUTS

Training Adaptation _____ Training Day_____

Exercise	Weight	Sets	Repetitions	Rest Interval

Notes _____

_____

_____

_____

"Fighting, to me, seems barbaric. I don't really like it. I enjoy out-thinking another man and out-maneuvering him, but I still don't like to fight."
—Sugar Ray Robinson

DAILY PLANNING: INDIVIDUAL WORKOUTS

Training Adaptation _____   Training Day_____

Exercise	Weight	Sets	Repetitions	Rest Interval

Notes

_____

_____

_____

Weekly Training

Training Phase _____

Mon	Tue	Wed	Thur	Fri	Sat	Sun

Training Modality	Method, Duration, Focus, Day(s)
Technical/Tactical	
Anaerobic	
Aerobic	
Resistance	

Notes

_____

_____

_____

_____

*"Let men see, let them know, a real man, who lives
as he was meant to live."*
—Marcus Aurelius

DAILY PLANNING: INDIVIDUAL WORKOUTS

Training Adaptation _____   Training Day _____

Exercise	Weight	Sets	Repetitions	Rest Interval

Notes

_____

_____

_____

"Greet what arrives, escort what leaves and
rush upon loss of contact."
—*Yip Man*

DAILY PLANNING: INDIVIDUAL WORKOUTS

Training Adaptation _____ Training Day_____

Exercise	Weight	Sets	Repetitions	Rest Interval

Notes

_____

_____

_____

"Passive inactivity, because you have not been given specific instructions to do this or to do that, is a serious deficiency."
—George C. Marshall

DAILY PLANNING: INDIVIDUAL WORKOUTS

Training Adaptation _____ Training Day_____

Exercise	Weight	Sets	Repetitions	Rest Interval

Notes
_____
_____
_____

"I may be kindly, I am ordinarily gentle, but in my line of business I am obliged to will terribly what I will at all."
—Catherine the Great

DAILY PLANNING: INDIVIDUAL WORKOUTS

Training Adaptation _____   Training Day_____

Exercise	Weight	Sets	Repetitions	Rest Interval

Notes
_____
_____
_____

"What you have been taught by listening to others' words you will forget very quickly; what you have learned with your whole body you will remember for the rest of your life."
—*Gichin Funakoshi*

DAILY PLANNING: INDIVIDUAL WORKOUTS

Training Adaptation _____   Training Day_____

Exercise	Weight	Sets	Repetitions	Rest Interval

Notes

_____
_____
_____

Weekly Training

Training Phase _____

Mon	Tue	Wed	Thur	Fri	Sat	Sun

Training Modality	Method, Duration, Focus, Day(s)
Technical/Tactical	
Anaerobic	
Aerobic	
Resistance	

Notes

_____

_____

_____

_____

"No one is so brave that he is not disturbed by
something unexpected."
—Julius Caesar

DAILY PLANNING: INDIVIDUAL WORKOUTS

Training Adaptation _____   Training Day _____

Exercise	Weight	Sets	Repetitions	Rest Interval

Notes
_____
_____
_____

"Talent and genius operate outside the rules, and theory conflicts with practice."
—Carl von Clausewitz

DAILY PLANNING: INDIVIDUAL WORKOUTS

Training Adaptation _____ Training Day_____

Exercise	Weight	Sets	Repetitions	Rest Interval

Notes

_____

_____

_____

"Vision without action is a daydream. Action with without vision is a nightmare."
—*Japanese proverb*

DAILY PLANNING: INDIVIDUAL WORKOUTS

Training Adaptation _____   Training Day_____

Exercise	Weight	Sets	Repetitions	Rest Interval

Notes

_____

_____

_____

"Come and take them."
—Leonidas I (In response to a demand from Xerxes I of Persia that the Spartans lay down their arms, at the Battle of Thermopylae.)

DAILY PLANNING: INDIVIDUAL WORKOUTS

Training Adaptation _____   Training Day_____

Exercise	Weight	Sets	Repetitions	Rest Interval

Notes
_____
_____
_____

"From one thing, know ten thousand things."

—*Miyamoto Musashi*

DAILY PLANNING: INDIVIDUAL WORKOUTS

Training Adaptation _____   Training Day_____

Exercise	Weight	Sets	Repetitions	Rest Interval

Notes _____

_____

_____

_____

Weekly Training

Training Phase _____

Mon	Tue	Wed	Thur	Fri	Sat	Sun

Training Modality	Method, Duration, Focus, Day(s)
Technical/Tactical	
Anaerobic	
Aerobic	
Resistance	

Notes

_____

_____

_____

_____

"It never troubles the wolf how many the sheep may be."

—Virgil

DAILY PLANNING: INDIVIDUAL WORKOUTS

Training Adaptation _____ Training Day_____

Exercise	Weight	Sets	Repetitions	Rest Interval

Notes

_____

_____

_____

"Any moment might be our last. Everything is more beautiful because we're doomed. You will never be lovelier than you are now. We will never be here again."
—Homer

DAILY PLANNING: INDIVIDUAL WORKOUTS

Training Adaptation _____   Training Day _____

Exercise	Weight	Sets	Repetitions	Rest Interval

Notes _____

_____

_____

_____

"It is monstrous that the feet should direct the head."

—*Elizabeth I*

DAILY PLANNING: INDIVIDUAL WORKOUTS

Training Adaptation _____ Training Day_____

Exercise	Weight	Sets	Repetitions	Rest Interval

Notes

_____

_____

_____

"Carefully observe oneself and one's situation, carefully observe others, and carefully observe one's environment. Consider fully, act decisively."
—Kano Jigoro

DAILY PLANNING: INDIVIDUAL WORKOUTS

Training Adaptation _____ Training Day_____

Exercise	Weight	Sets	Repetitions	Rest Interval

Notes
_____
_____
_____

"I spent my life—all my life—learning to wrestle. It's the only means of livelihood I've ever had, and uh, the only gimmick I have in wrestling is wrestling."
—Gene Lebbell

DAILY PLANNING: INDIVIDUAL WORKOUTS

Training Adaptation _____   Training Day_____

Exercise	Weight	Sets	Repetitions	Rest Interval

Notes _____

_____

_____

Weekly Training

Training Phase _____

Mon	Tue	Wed	Thur	Fri	Sat	Sun

Training Modality	Method, Duration, Focus, Day(s)
Technical/Tactical	
Anaerobic	
Aerobic	
Resistance	

Notes

_____

_____

_____

_____

"With uncertainty in one scale, courage and self-confidence should be thrown into the other to correct the balance. The greater they are, the greater the margin that can be left for accidents."
—Carl von Clausewitz

DAILY PLANNING: INDIVIDUAL WORKOUTS

Training Adaptation _____ Training Day_____

Exercise	Weight	Sets	Repetitions	Rest Interval

Notes

_____

_____

_____

"Progress comes to those who train and train; reliance on secret techniques will get you nowhere."
—*Morihei Ueshiba*

DAILY PLANNING: INDIVIDUAL WORKOUTS

Training Adaptation _____   Training Day_____

Exercise	Weight	Sets	Repetitions	Rest Interval

Notes

_____

_____

_____

"A mind not to be changed by place or time. The mind is its own place, and in itself can make a heaven of hell, a hell of heaven."
—*Milton*

DAILY PLANNING: INDIVIDUAL WORKOUTS

Training Adaptation _____   Training Day_____

Exercise	Weight	Sets	Repetitions	Rest Interval

Notes

_____

_____

_____

"The greater the difficulty, the more the glory in surmounting it."

—Epicurus

DAILY PLANNING: INDIVIDUAL WORKOUTS

Training Adaptation _____   Training Day_____

Exercise	Weight	Sets	Repetitions	Rest Interval

Notes
_____

_____

_____

_____

"You can only fight the way you practice."

—Miyamoto Musashi

DAILY PLANNING: INDIVIDUAL WORKOUTS

Training Adaptation _____   Training Day_____

Exercise	Weight	Sets	Repetitions	Rest Interval

Notes

_____

_____

_____

Weekly Training

Training Phase _____

Mon	Tue	Wed	Thur	Fri	Sat	Sun

Training Modality	Method, Duration, Focus, Day(s)
Technical/Tactical	
Anaerobic	
Aerobic	
Resistance	

Notes

_____

_____

_____

_____

"Victory belongs to the most persevering."

—Napoleon

DAILY PLANNING: INDIVIDUAL WORKOUTS

Training Adaptation _____   Training Day_____

Exercise	Weight	Sets	Repetitions	Rest Interval

Notes
_____
_____
_____

"Men become builders by building and lyre players by playing the lyre; so too we become just by doing just acts, temperate by doing temperate acts, brave by doing brave acts."
—*Aristotle*

DAILY PLANNING: INDIVIDUAL WORKOUTS

Training Adaptation _____ Training Day_____

Exercise	Weight	Sets	Repetitions	Rest Interval

Notes

_____

_____

_____

"It is difficult for a student to pick a good teacher, but it is more difficult for a teacher to pick a good student."
—Yip Man

DAILY PLANNING: INDIVIDUAL WORKOUTS

Training Adaptation _____   Training Day_____

Exercise	Weight	Sets	Repetitions	Rest Interval

Notes
_____
_____
_____
_____

"I can show you how to box. I can teach you every technique and trick I know, but I can never make you a fighter. That comes from inside, and it's something no one else can ever give you."
—Joe Louis

DAILY PLANNING: INDIVIDUAL WORKOUTS

Training Adaptation _____   Training Day _____

Exercise	Weight	Sets	Repetitions	Rest Interval

Notes _____

_____

_____

_____

*"Every suspension of offensive action, either from erroneous views,
from fear or from indolence, is in favor of the side acting defensively."*
—Carl von Clausewitz

DAILY PLANNING: INDIVIDUAL WORKOUTS

Training Adaptation _____   Training Day_____

Exercise	Weight	Sets	Repetitions	Rest Interval

Notes
_____
_____
_____

Weekly Training

Training Phase _____

Mon	Tue	Wed	Thur	Fri	Sat	Sun

Training Modality	Method, Duration, Focus, Day(s)
Technical/Tactical	
Anaerobic	
Aerobic	
Resistance	

Notes

_____
_____
_____
_____

"Impossible is a word only to be found in the lexicon of fools."

—Napoleon

DAILY PLANNING: INDIVIDUAL WORKOUTS

Training Adaptation _____   Training Day_____

Exercise	Weight	Sets	Repetitions	Rest Interval

Notes
_____
_____
_____

"Once that bell rings you're on your own.
It's just you and the other guy."
—Joe Louis

DAILY PLANNING: INDIVIDUAL WORKOUTS

Training Adaptation _____   Training Day_____

Exercise	Weight	Sets	Repetitions	Rest Interval

Notes _____
_____
_____
_____

"Then imitate the action of the tiger; stiffen the sinews, summon up the blood."
—*William Shakespeare*

DAILY PLANNING: INDIVIDUAL WORKOUTS

Training Adaptation _____   Training Day_____

Exercise	Weight	Sets	Repetitions	Rest Interval

Notes _____

_____

_____

_____

"When two tigers fight, one is certain to be maimed, and one to die."

—*Gichin Funakoshi*

DAILY PLANNING: INDIVIDUAL WORKOUTS

Training Adaptation _____   Training Day_____

Exercise	Weight	Sets	Repetitions	Rest Interval

Notes _____

_____

_____

_____

"The art of living is more like wrestling than dancing."

—Marcus Aurelius

DAILY PLANNING: INDIVIDUAL WORKOUTS

Training Adaptation _____   Training Day_____

Exercise	Weight	Sets	Repetitions	Rest Interval

Notes
_____
_____
_____

WHAT TYPE OF FIGHTER ARE YOU?

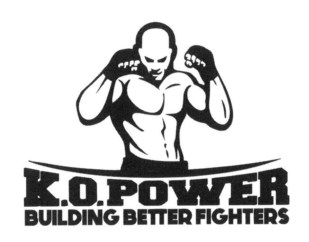

As you well know, not all fighters are alike, and their differences go beyond stylistic differences such as in-fighter or out-fighter; virtuoso boxer or brawler, striker or grappler, but is related to your core temperament. Your temperament could be said to be a configuration of psychological characteristics, inclinations and patterns of action. Temperament also includes your individual goals and determines your preferred way of achieving them.

Coach Mark Ginther has adapted the historical concept of 4 distinct temperaments, classifying them as: the Warrior, the Solider, the General and the Paladin.

Take the following quiz (adapted from David Keirsey's Temperament Sorter) to learn which kind of fighter you are, along with your particular strengths and weaknesses. Consider each question and number answers 1–4 depending on how closely they describe you (1 for most; 4 for least).

1. I feel best about my training when:

   A. My movements are fluid and effortless.
   B. There is a positive 'vibe' in the gym/dojo atmosphere
   C. I strictly adhere to my schedule (no missed workouts, etc.)
   D. My training is productive and efficient

2. I am drawn to martial arts and combat-sports for:

   A. Visceral excitement and fun
   B. A journey of self-discovery
   C. To protect self and loved ones
   D. To expand my physical prowess.

3. If I were to become famous as a martial artist or fighter I'd use my fame to:

A. Go into action films
B. Use my knowledge and wisdom to help others become their best selves
C. Open a chain of gyms bearing my name
D. Market my unique and specialized training system

4. The greatest appeal of the traditional martial arts is:

A. Their use of weaponry
B. Their wisdom and spirituality
C. Their rich history and tradition
D. Their knowledge of the arcane and esoteric

5. The most important factor in determining success in a fight or match is:

A. Skills
B. Self-knowledge
C. Training
D. Planning

6. In training I emphasize:

A. Developing my abilities
B. Self-discovery and improvement
C. Self-discipline and correct technique
D. Identifying and using the core principles behind the sport/system

7. In the ring or on the mat, I am most inclined to follow:

A. My gut
B. My heart
C. My experience and training
D. My game-plan/strategy

8. In the dojo or gym I want to:

  A. Make a strong impact on other members
  B. Be a mentor to other members
  C. Be a valued and legitimate member
  D. Find a better more efficient way to do things

9. I am pleased when students or training partners:

  A. Are generous with their time/knowledge
  B. Seek me out for my council/wisdom
  C. Show their appreciation for my support and effort
  D. Ask me for my input and analysis

10. Which of the following action movie characters do you relate to the most?

  A. James Bond/007 in *Skyfall*, Wade Wilson/Deadpool in *Deadpool*, Django Freeman in *Django Unchained*
  B. Neo in *The Matrix*, Luke Skywalker in *Star Wars*, Thor in *The Avengers*,
  C. Judge Dredd in *Dredd*, Steve Rogers/Captain America in *The Avengers*, Kal El/Superman in *The Man of Steel*
  D. V in *V for Vendetta*, Tony Stark/Iron Man in *The Avengers*, Dr. Jonathan Osterman/Dr. Manhattan in *Watchmen*

11. The aspect of martial arts or combat-sports I am most interested in developing is:

  A. Technical and tactical abilities
  B. Philosophical, psychological and spiritual aspects
  C. Mental and physical discipline
  D. Core principles and strategies

12. When facing loss or defeat, my attitude tends to be:

  A. Tomorrow is another day.
  B. Why?
  C. Get up; soldier on.
  D. How does this affect my grand strategy?

13. In achieving my goals I tend (or try) to be

  A. Practical and opportunistic
  B. Humane and altruistic
  C. Diligent and dutiful
  D. Efficient and pragmatic

14. When fighting or sparring I am most confident when:

  A. I am in the 'zone'
  B. At peace with myself and my opponent
  C. My coach and corner have my back
  D. I have a solid game-plan

15. When considering the future of my career:

  A. Something will turn up, it always does
  B. You should follow your bliss
  C. I had better prepare a 'safety-net'
  D. I always have a contingency plan

16. I have the most self-respect when I am:

  A. Bold and courageous
  B. Altruistic and compassionate
  C. I am a rock, an anchor for friends and teammates
  D. I am autonomous and self-reliant

17. People who dislike or don't know me well might describe me as:

A. Impulsive, self-centered
B. Flakey, quixotic
C. Stubborn, dogmatic
D. Cold, arrogant

18. When coaching or instructing I tend to emphasize:

A. Demonstration of technique
B. Promoting a harmonious atmosphere
C. Discipline and hard work
D. A logical, systematic approach

19. When sparring or fighting another opponent I try to:

A. Overcome them with superior tactics and abilities
B. Act appropriately and proportionately to their actions
C. Overcome them with courage and tenacity
D. Out-think and out maneuver them

20. The quote I identify with most is:

A. "Lead me, follow me, or get out of my way." —George S. Patton
B. "Nine-tenths of tactics are certain, and taught in books: but the irrational tenth is like the kingfisher flashing across the pool, and that is the test of generals." —T.E. Lawrence
C. "Discipline strengthens the mind so that it becomes impervious to the corroding influence of fear." —Bernard Montgomery
D. "Strength of character does not consist solely of having powerful feelings, but maintaining one's balance in spite of them." —Carl von Clausewitz

Tally your scores and determine which answers, A, B, C or D you chose number 1 for most often. If most of your answers identify with—

A, you are **THE WARRIOR**

B, you are **THE PALADIN**

C, you are **THE SOLDIER**

D, you are **THE GENERAL**

Descriptions and analysis follow here:

THE WARRIOR

You are a natural-born fighter. Like a musician that can play by ear, you don't need to be taught skills, just shown and you 'get' it. Those of you that are able to combine your natural talents with good coaching and hard work, often become legends of the sport —the best of the best, the greatest, and other such epithets adorn many of your type. Bold, unconventional, and spontaneous. You live in the moment, which is an asset in the ring, cage or on the mat, as you react to whatever is thrown at you without reservation. You can 'roll with the punches' and make the best of any situation. You like fighting for the sake of fighting, the thrill of combat, the rush of adrenaline, and the heightened senses make you feel alive. You are a skilled tactician that does what needs to be done at the moment.

In training you are not concerned with tradition so much as with what works in the here and now. Bruce Lee's famous motto, 'Absorb what is useful, reject what is useful' exemplifies your approach to training. You may be impatient with structured lessons and classes, preferring to do your own thing, either training alone or friends of a similar level. You also have little time for theory and principles, save that for the Generals, you just want to get into the action.

In competition, you are likely to be as much showman as athlete, whether your persona is loud and flamboyant or quiet and brooding, golden boy or heel, the crowd will be drawn to your innate charisma, and will always be a crowd-pleaser. You tend to trust your gut, and are bold and optimistic, willing to stand toe-to-toe with a strong opponent and throw down, toss the dice, as it were.

The majority high-level professional fighters are of your type.

Strengths: Adaptable, creative, competitive; willing to take risks.

Weaknesses: Impulsive, even rash. May have trouble sticking to a game-plan, or listening to your corner. Fighters that are called 'un-coachable' are usually of this type.

In the terms of the ancient Roman physician, Galen, your type corresponds to the temperament, Sanguine.

THE SOLDIER

You are a formidable fighter that is driven by a strong sense of duty and service, be it to family, teammates or a principle. You are a traditionalist, the warhorse, old-guard, a professional. You are a loyal member of the team, and seek a strong sense of belonging with the members of your gym, dojo or club. Though lacking the natural gifts of 'The Warrior', you can often make up for this with your strong work ethic, and drive In the gym or dojo you are highly respectful to your teachers and seniors, and you demand respect from those below you in rank or experience.

In training you take a serious, no-nonsense approach, you are reliable and unlikely to skip workouts, and are respectful of your teachers or coaches and dutifully follow their instructions. You take the long-term approach and don't rush or cut corners (slow and steady wins the race).

In competition you tend to trust and rely on your past experiences. Your strong work ethic and sense of duty can make you a daunting opponent, however your biggest weakness may be inflexibility. You may find it difficult to adapt to circumstances, preferring to stick with what you do best, even if it isn't working in a given situation. You can however overcome this if you have a good coach/corner, and listen them.

Strengths: Strong work ethic, stoic, highly coachable, long-term goal setting.

Weaknesses: Inflexibility, stubbornness, overly risk-adverse.

In the terms of the ancient Roman physician, Galen, your type corresponds to the temperament, Melancholic.

THE PALADIN

You are the Shaolin Monks and Jedi Knights of the fight world, the champions of noble causes. Your interest in martial arts and/or fight-sports is part of your quest towards greater personal growth and development. You are more likely to be drawn the traditional martial arts than fight-sports because of their philosophical and spiritual aspects (especially those such as tai chi or aikido), and use them as part of your never-ending search for self-knowledge. You have a sage-like quality and often appear wise beyond your years. As a coach, instructor or training partner you are devoted to helping others be their best selves.

In training you are interested in developing the psychological and spiritual aspects as much, or more so than the physical skills, and are likely to engage in meditation or similar practices. You tend to cooperate with, rather than compete against your training partners, as you are concerned not only with your own progress, but with your classmates and teammates as well.

As a competitor you are less likely to let your pride and ego get in the way than the other types, allowing you to react more naturally to whatever comes. Your greatest weakness may be that you are as likely to feel bad for a beaten opponent as take pleasure and pride in your victory, which may cause you to hold back rather than finishing an opponent.

Strengths: Imaginative, intuitive, adaptable, wise

Weaknesses: Lacking a killer-instinct (only a weakness in combat-sport competition).

In the terms of the ancient Roman physician, Galen, your type corresponds to the temperament, Choleric.

THE GENERAL

You are logical, rational, and analytical. Though lacking the tactical, roll-with-the-punches, abilities of the Warrior, you have the greatest strategic abilities of all the types. This serves you well when devising a game-plan against a known opponent, as does your ability to quickly and accurately identify weaknesses in your opponent's offense and defense. You are ruthlessly pragmatic and will do what is necessary to beat your opponent. More than any of the other types you are likely to be interested in the science and theory behind training and fighting and therefore will often make a better coach than competitor.

In training you take a problem-solving approach, and rather than just putting in long hours and hard work, you look for the most time and energy efficient ways achieving your goals. You are likely to follow the old adage, 'less is more'.

In competition, you will stick to your game-plan and be systematic about picking apart your opponent. However, if forced from your game-plan, you may have trouble adapting to circumstances, and will need to listen to your coach/corner to get out of trouble. Though not risk-adverse, you prefer playing chess to throwing dice (i.e. brawling). You take the Sun Tzu approach: You won't accept battle (take a fight) unless you've already won (completely sure that you will be victorious).

Strengths: Logical, systematic, big-picture oriented, cool-headed.

Weaknesses: Analysis-paralysis, reluctance to risk a loss.

In the terms of the ancient Roman physician, Galen, your type corresponds to the temperament, Phlegmatic

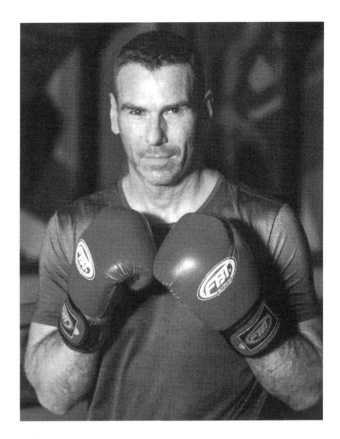

ABOUT MARK GINTHER, COACH & AUTHOR

Mark Ginther is a martial artist, former competitive kickboxer, fight coach, strength & conditioning coach and author with over 35 years' experience.

Mark has trained and sparred with some of the greats, including UFC champion, Maurice Smith at the original AMC Kickboxing, later becoming the strength coach for the new AMC Kickboxing & Pankration under Matt Hume, as well as (stand-up) sparring partner for future UFC champion, Josh Barnett.

Mark has coached top professional and amateur fighters in the USA, Japan and Thailand (including UFC heavyweight contender, Mark Hunt), and has written for many of the top publications in the industry. His book, *K.O. Power: Complete Strength Training for Devastating Punches, Kicks & Throws* has been on the Amazon Bestsellers list for Mixed Martial Arts, Boxing and Martial Arts for over a year (often in the top ten and reaching #6 in MMA and #4 in Boxing).

In Japan, Mark was the strength & conditioning coach, kickboxing coach and corner man for Athletic Enterprise; training such fighters as Mark Hunt, Peter Graham, Nicholas Pettas and Bob Sapp. While in Japan he also began writing a long-running strength & conditioning column for *Full Contact Fighter*, which was reprinted in Japanese in *Ironman Japan*.

In Thailand, Mark was the head striking coach at Bangkok Fight Lab, heading the boxing program, teaching K-1 rules kickboxing and providing striking coaching for MMA fighters. In the one year he spent at Fight Lab, seven of his boxers competed in a total of 13 fights, with 11 wins, 2 draws, and 0 losses.

Mark also help launch The Hook Boxing Gym, the first ever boxing gym in Kuwait, where he coached boxing, kickboxing, and strength & conditioning.

After nearly 20 years training and coaching abroad, Mark has returned to his home base in the USA, where he is currently striking coach at West Coast Fight Team in Auburn, Washington.

Made in the USA
Lexington, KY
17 January 2019